A LESSON IN DYING

By Nathan Harrison

Copyright © 2025 Nathan Harrison

All rights reserved.

ISBN:

Dedication

To all those fighting the same or similar battle.

To the scared children who think they are forgotten.

To the family members who watch the suffering and don't know what to do. To my family, my departed mother, my friends whose names I often struggle with, the stranger I'll never meet.

This is for you. This is for us.

Preface

This book is for all of us.

For the warrior who now struggles to lift his own hand
once strong, unshakable, now brought low by time or illness,
but still fighting with everything he has left.

For the soft-hearted child the world tried to break
the one who was forced to grow up too soon,
who turned pain into purpose and scars into strength.

For the wife who sits quietly beside her husband,

holding his hand as she prepares to say goodbye
her love steady, even when her heart is breaking.

For the husband who wants to make sure his love is known,
his legacy clear,
his final words filled with meaning and truth.
A man who may be dying
but refuses to leave without saying what matters most.

This book is for anyone walking through the fire
the caregiver, the patient, the child watching a parent fade.
For those who whisper prayers in hospital rooms

and hold on to hope even when the world
says to let go.

I wrote this not just as a farewell,
but as a hand reaching out in the dark
to say you're not alone.

I am fighting with you.
I am standing beside you in spirit.
And I pray truly that you find the peace
you deserve.

Not just in the end,
but in the moments before it,
and in the love that will carry on long
after we're gone.

Table of Contents
1. A Lesson in Dying
2. The Quiet War
3. What I Leave Behind
4. Memory and the Mind
5. The Measure of a Man
6. Carrying the Lost
7. Words You Need To Hear
8. Stories I'll Never Tell
9. What I've Learned from Dying
10. When the Dew Settles

Chapter One: A Lesson in Dying

Poem: This Pain I Carry
"I carry pain like a badge, not of honor, but of truth,
Etched into marrow, in defiance of my youth.
It whispers at night when the morphine stays sealed,
A voice from the past that never quite healed.

I ache and I falter, but still I remain,
Chained to the memories, humbled by pain.
Not begging for mercy, not asking for fame
Just hoping my children will remember my name."

You ever sat beside someone you love as they lay dying? I mean really sat. Quiet. No phone, no clock-watching, no small talk to fill the air. Just stillness Watching their eyes drift not closed, not gone, just… somewhere far off. Someplace you can't follow. And in that silence between each breath, you find yourself wondering what they're thinking. Wondering if they're holding on for you, or if they've already started letting go. You search for words, but none feel right. You wonder if there's something they need to hear or maybe something they're trying to teach you. Some secret, some wisdom, wrapped in the stillness of those final moments. A lesson, maybe, in dying.

"Do you have an end-of-life plan?" The doctor didn't whisper it. Didn't soften it with a pause or glance or even a sigh. Just cut straight through the quiet like a blade across frostbitten skin. And I've carried that sentence ever since. Echoed it in my head on long nights and longer mornings. Not because he meant harm, but because there's no soft way to say something like that. Some truths come sharp, whether you're ready or not. There's a moment; quiet, unannounced when dying becomes more than an idea. It slips past the textbooks and doctors, past the polite phrases and casseroles left on the porch. One day you're just tired, the next you're watching the hands on the clock and wondering how many more turns they've got left. Dying isn't always sudden. Sometimes, it's slow as rust and twice as cruel. I didn't learn about death in a hospital bed. I learned about it in the field: military and police both, watching it steal fathers and sons, wives and children, good folks and bad ones, without asking permission or offering explanation. I've seen it come with a whisper, and I've seen it come with a scream. And now, it's coming for me. You don't think about the act of dying until it becomes your job. My job, for a while now, has been to die. To do it slowly. To try to do it with some kind of grace. To leave a trail my children can follow, not one paved in sorrow, but in meaning. And let me tell you something most folks won't: dying teaches you more about living than all the living ever did. Pain becomes your preacher. Regret becomes your schoolmaster. And if you're lucky, love becomes your compass. I've hurt in ways I can't describe. Physically, sure but the emotional toll? That's the one that knocks the breath out of you on the days when you're already gasping. I've had to watch my kids carry the weight of seeing their daddy fade. That isn't something a father ever wants. I've had to sit across from my wife and pretend I'm not scared, not hurting, not breaking inside. I've had to say goodbye in a thousand small ways, hoping they won't remember me as weak or pitiful, but as a man who kept fighting, even when the war turned inward. This chapter isn't just about dying it's about preparing. About leaving nothing unsaid. About carving a trail so those I love can walk it long after I'm gone. If you're reading this, chances are you're either dying or loving someone who is. And I need you to hear me: you are not alone. The silence, the shame, the slow decay none of it means you're weak. None of it makes you less. It makes you human. I wrote this not as a man who gave up, but as a man who looked death in the eyes and said, "Not today. Not until I've finished my story." And this story? It's not about the end. It's about the fight to finish with meaning. About teaching my kids what matters while I still can. About making peace with the man, I was, and the man I hope they'll remember. I don't know how many pages I have left. But I'll write until my hands give out, and when they do, I hope these words linger like footprints in wet clay faded, maybe, but still leading somewhere. Somewhere good.

Let me tell you what dying feels like. It isn't silence. It's a storm that rattles the windows of your soul, but only you can hear it. The house stays still; the trees don't sway but inside? Inside, the wind howls through everything you ever were

But not all of them.

My VA doctor, Natalie, she came at it different. From day one, she brought more than medicine. She brought warmth. There's something sacred about a woman who can speak the hard truths but still leave you feeling comforted. She never looked at me like a case file. She saw the man beneath the diagnosis. And I'll carry gratitude for her as long as I've got breath to carry anything.

Amanda Fisher was another light in the early dark. When I didn't have the words, she waited. When I didn't know the questions to ask, she gave me answers that felt like grace. They didn't just treat symptoms. They treated and helped me.

These days, it's my hospice team keeping the storm at bay. Kat. Angel. And the rest of the crew. Women with hands steady as old trees and hearts kind enough to weather any sorrow. There's a strange kind of grace in how life loops back on itself. Full circles, hidden threads things you don't see coming until they're already wrapped around your heart.

Kim Holly was the police chief when I left the department. He was tough, fair, and steady the kind of leader that didn't have to shout to be respected. I remember how he carried himself, how he backed his people, how he never asked anyone to do something he wouldn't do himself.

And now, years later, his daughter Samantha walks through the door of my home as one of my hospice nurses.

Let that settle in.

The child of a chief who once helped shepherd my career… now helping shepherd me to the end of mine. But it doesn't feel like an ending, not with her or with any of my nurses. It feels like being cared for by someone who understands where I've been even if they didn't walk those halls themselves.

They're gentle but firm. The kind of women who listens more than they speaks. Who knows when to talk, when to just sit, and when a hand on your arm means more than anything you could say out loud.

Sometimes when they're checking vitals or adjusting my meds, I catch myself thinking how proud her daddy must be. Different badge, same kind of courage.

It's a quiet, full-circle kind of beauty. And it reminds me:

We never really leave behind the good we do. It just comes back, sometimes years later, wearing scrubs instead of a uniform, holding a stethoscope instead of a clipboard… but carrying the same kind of strength all the same.
They don't just come to ease pain. They come to remind me: I'm still human. Still seen. Still loved. They don't flinch when I cry. They don't rush the hard moments. They bring dignity with them like it's packed in their nurse's bag right next to the morphine. They show up day after day like it matters. Because to them, it does.

I hurt.

Some days, it feels like my bones are screaming. There's medicine that'll dull it, but I don't take it the way I should. Maybe that's pride. Maybe fear. I spent too many years cuffing addicts watching pills steal men's names, watching powders burn bridges that love couldn't rebuild. And now I sit here wondering if I'll fall down that same hole
right at the end. Or maybe, just maybe, I want to keep my mind sharp. Even if the blade's chipped and rusted I still want to hold it steady in my own hands. Or maybe I feel like I deserve the pain. Old sins circling back like hounds. And this hurt? It's penance. So, I let the pain stay. Let it walk beside me like an old friend I can't shake. Lord, some days I swear the pain could split me clean in half. I've got medicine sitting right beside me. Stuff I'm supposed to take more often. Strong

enough to knock the edge off. But I don't. But the truth is I want to stay clear. My mind might be cracked, but what pieces remain, I want to feel them. Hold them close. So, I grit my teeth and live with the pain. That, too, is a kind of faith. My mind doesn't rest. Never has. It loops like an old Super 8, grainy and stubborn, memories I wish I could scrub clean, moments I'd trade my last breath to walk through again, words I never said out loud, but whispered too late to matter. My mind never quiets. It runs in circles some days chasing regrets, some days chasing ghosts. Memories I'd give anything to rewrite. Futures I know I won't see.

I lay here dreaming of days that may never come. Making plans for when I feel better. And when I do feel better? I'm still here. Still lying still. Still fading. I remember my mama, when hospice had

her in its grip. Planning mountain trips, knowing full well she'd never drive the Cades Cove again. And now look at me. Talking about fixing fence lines and hunting trips that'll never happen. I ought to know better. But hope… hope is a wild thing. It doesn't die easy. Let that be your first lesson. Hope is the last light to leave a man. I used to wonder why.
Now I understand.

Hope is the last thing a dying person lets go of. And next to love, it's the greatest thing we've got.

I've sat with dying men before. Soldiers. Suspects. Family. Back then, I wondered what they were thinking in those final breaths. Were they scared? Were they at peace? Were they angry? Did they regret? Now I know. It's all of it. At once.
Love and shame, peace and panic, clarity and confusion. The mind opens wide in

the end. You think about who you loved. And who you failed.
You remember the birthdays you missed, the arguments that should've ended with a hug, the mornings you should've said I love you instead of hurry up. You think about your children. And how they'll remember you. You hope to God they'll remember more than the dying.
You hope they hear your voice in their hearts long after it's gone from this world.
  This book… is my voice. It's what I leave behind. I don't want pity. I want presence. I want my son to know: Real strength isn't in hiding pain it's in standing through it. And I want my daughter to know: Love isn't earned. It's lived. Loudly. Boldly. Without apology. There's a difference between dying and quitting. I may be dying. But I ain't quitting. I write this for my wife. My

babies. My people. And I write it for strangers who may never know my name, but who walk a path that feels like mine.

This ain't just a story. It's a testimony. Of what it feels like when your body betrays you. When your mind slips away in pieces. When pain becomes a roommate, you never invited but can't evict. But it's also about more. It's about the people who show up anyway.

Who hold your hand when you can't hold a spoon. Who love you through the mess and the morphine. Who remind you that even when your flesh is failing your soul still shines.

This is what it means to live while dying. To fade but still feel. To hurt but still hope. To fear but still choose love. Because there's wisdom in dying. If you listen for it. It teaches you not just how to let go but how we should've been living all along. If you're sick If you're the one lying in that bed hear me: You are not alone. Even in the silence. Even in the ache. You are still worthy. Still needed. Still loved. And if you're the one standing by the bed wiping the brow, whispering I'm here, fighting tears in the hallway You are holy. The world may not see it, but I do. And so does the one you're loving through their final breath. This isn't a goodbye. This is a companion. A voice for the sleepless nights. A hand on your back when no one else understands. A reminder that even now there is beauty. There is meaning. There is connection. This book is my way of saying: We're in this together. Now I'll tell you the truth

   Some of this might not read clean. It may ramble. It may jump around like a memory caught in a storm. That's because it's real. I've written and rewritten these

pages more times than I can count.
Sometimes the words slipped away before
I could catch them. Sometimes my mind
betrayed me before the sentence could
settle. I thought about hiring someone to
make it pretty. But dying ain't pretty.
And this ain't supposed to be either. It's
real. And sometimes real is raw, and
messy, and hard to follow. But if you've
ever walked through hospice laid in that
bed or held the hand of someone who did
then you already understand the fog.
You understand the fear. The fight to
speak truth before time steals your voice.
This book may not be polished. But it is
honest. It is mine. And it is yours, now.
So, if you've made it this far,
maybe something in these pages will help
you understand the ones you love.
Maybe you'll hear them better.
Love them more deeply. Forgive faster.

Live fuller. And maybe just maybe you'll learn a little something about dying. And in that…you'll find a better way to live.

Chapter Two: The Quiet War

Poem: Silent Battles
"Not all wars echo with gunfire and cries,
Some are fought behind faraway eyes.
In a hospital bed or a memory's haze,
Where silence screams louder than battle displays. I carried my rifle, now I carry a cane,
Swapped my uniform for IVs and pain.
But don't call me weak don't say I'm done,
I'm still fighting battles that can't be outrun."

Most people don't understand the war that happens after the service. They see soldiers come home, badges retired, uniforms folded and put away like everything's finished. But the truth is the fight don't end. It just gets quiet. Quieter than most folks can hear. This kind of war ain't loud. There's no gunfire. No sirens. No screaming radios or crunch of boots. It's the hum of IV pumps and the soft click of a morphine button. It's the creak of the porch swing when your body hurts too bad to sit, but you're too proud to go inside. It's the look in your child's eyes when they ask if you're okay and you lie. Because you love them more than the truth. I used to wear armor. Real armor. Vest, badge, rifle. I've stormed doors with steel in my hands and prayers in my mouth. I've tracked evil through woods and back alleys, brought justice when no one else would. I was damn good at it. Maybe too good. But now? Now I fight a war that don't give medals. No ceremony. No victory lap. It's me, an old bed, and time and she's a ruthless enemy. You want to know what dying feels like? It's not just pain. It's powerlessness. Watching your body shrink. Watching your family tiptoe around your moods because they don't know if it's pain or grief making you cold that day. It's hearing your name said soft, like it might break you. Like you might break. It's people asking how they can help, and you don't know what to say, because what you really want, they can't give: your health, your strength, your life back. But you smile. You say thank you. Because that's the kind of man you were raised to be.

I miss strange things. The weight of a duty belt on my hips.
The burn in my thighs after a long day cutting firewood. The quiet walk-through early morning fields, dew soaking my boots, heart listening for movement in the trees. I miss being needed. Being called. I

miss that split second when instinct took over and I didn't have to think just act. Just move. Just be. You don't realize how much of your identity is tied to what your body can still do. Until it can't. And in all that stillness,
the mind gets loud. I lie here, and everything comes back. The children I tried to save. The ones I couldn't.
The good men I worked besides, some still living, some not. The nights I got home too late to kiss my baby's goodnight. The morning coffee left cold while I wrote one more report. The things I sacrificed, thinking I had more time. God, I thought I had more time.

  People talk about bravery like it only lives in bullets and battlefields. But I've found a different kind of courage now. It's in getting up when every part of you aches. It's in smiling at your daughter when she paints your toenails pink just to make you laugh. It's in letting people care for you, even when your pride hates it. It's in saying I'm scared and not following it with an apology. Because this war: this quiet war it takes everything you got and then dares you to give more I think about my kids.

What they'll remember. Will they remember the man I was at my strongest, or the man who held on even when he was at his weakest? Will they know the cost I paid to protect them?

Will they know that I never stopped being their father, even when I could no longer carry them? That I never stopped fighting even when the war went silent?

   The battlefield has changed. The armor's gone. But I'm still a warrior. I fight every single day. For peace. For presence. For one more sunrise. So, if you're walking through your own quiet war whether it's sickness or sorrow or something you can't even name Know this: You're not alone. I see you. I am you. And even now, even here…I'm still fighting.

There's a war going on inside me, and most days no one sees it. When I served, I wore the uniform, kept my boots clean, and followed orders. I trained hard. I stood shoulder to shoulder with men who would've died for me, and I for them. And when I got hurt, really hurt, part of that came home with me. Except now the enemy doesn't wear a uniform. It hides in my muscles, my mind, my memory. The quiet war is the one nobody talks about.

My injury, a traumatic brain injury, didn't come with medals or a ceremony. It came with fog. It came with frustration. It came with forgetting names of people I love, losing time, losing thoughts mid-sentence. It came with whispers in the night and the shame of asking your child to remind you where you left your keys… again. You see, the quiet war doesn't make the news. No one salutes the man in the grocery store who stands there too long, trying to remember what he came in for. No one honors the dad who locks himself in the bathroom because he doesn't want his children to see him cry over a memory he can't explain. But we fight. Every day. And not just me. There are veterans, nurses, cops, kids, moms, people fighting quiet wars all over this world. Some scars you see. Others are buried so deep it takes courage just to wake up. I fought in the Army, then again as a police investigator. I saw things that would make most men fall apart and for a long time, I didn't fall apart. I just packed it all down, like carrying an extra magazine of ammo. Just in case. Just in case I needed the pain. Just in case the rage kept me sharp. That works… until it doesn't. The real war didn't begin until I was alone with my thoughts. Until I lost my job, my health, and the illusion that I could fix everything. That's when you start measuring your life in minutes of clarity, hours without pain, and moments when your kids make you laugh, and you forget you're dying. That's what keeps me in the fight. Riley and Harper. My son and daughter. My reasons. They don't know how heavy my war is but one day, they will. And when they do, I want them to know their daddy didn't give up. He just ran out of time.

   First Sergeant Fraley told me once during a quiet phone call,
"Harrison, at some point you've got to be honest with yourself about what's

happening to you." His words hit harder than I expected because deep down, I already knew he was right. Just a few days before, I'd had a VA appointment in Memphis…but I got turned around, confused, and drove 70 miles in the wrong direction. My mind was slipping.

The doctors at Landstuhl had warned me this would happen, but I kept thinking I had more time. I wasn't ready for it to happen so soon. I had already stopped going out to eat at work,
because hiding my shaking hands was getting harder by the day. I remember sitting in CIPIT meetings stomach growling, being so hungry, but also being too embarrassed to eat. Too embarrassed to show my shaking hands, to show weakness. Yes, I was failing and soon, I'd have to stop pretending otherwise. There's a moment when you just know.

Even if no one else sees it, something deep inside you does a quiet, aching whisper in your bones telling you…your time is running out. Truthfully, if it hadn't been for First Sergeant Fraley and my section sergeant, SFC Maggard, I don't think I would've made it as long as I did in the army. SFC Maggard is more than a fellow soldier he's, my brother. He never mentioned my health out loud, never made me feel exposed, but he saw it before I did. While I was trying to hold it together, he quietly stepped in. He kept me off the radar always had me on some "detail," somewhere out of sight, out of mind. He was shielding me in the only way he could, and I'll always be grateful for that.

    I won't weigh this book down with army stories this isn't about my time in

the Army. This is something else. This is
a reference for the ones feeling lost,
a quiet guide for those standing at the
edge of the unknown, wondering what
comes next, or what words might matter
most. We all fight quiet wars. Battles that
rage behind the eyes, wars no one else can
see. We carry them tucked deep inside our
souls hidden beneath forced smiles, polite
answers, and the brave face we wear to
get through the day.

  We scream…but only on the inside.
The world sees calm, but inside there's a
storm tearing through everything familiar.
And we convince ourselves no one else
could possibly understand,
that if they knew what we were really
feeling, they'd walk away. But the truth is
we've all been there. Every one of us has
scars, some visible, most not. We've all

had nights where we stared at the ceiling, wondering if anyone would notice if we just stopped showing up.
We've all fought those moments where giving up felt easier than getting up. But here's what we must learn and it's not easy, but it's true: There is no shame in crying out for help. There is no weakness in needing someone to see you,
to hold your hand,
to simply say, "You're not alone." We must believe especially when it feels hardest to believe that we are worthy of love. Even when we feel broken. Even when we feel like a burden. Even when we've convinced ourselves we don't deserve it. Because we do. And not only that we're still capable of giving love. Of being light for someone else, even if our own world feels dim. We are silent warriors. But I hear your cries. I feel your

pain. I see your battle, even if no one else does. And if no one's told you lately I'm proud of you for holding on.

So let this be another lesson: Not strength. Not survival. Not endurance. But love. Because love is what makes any of this worth it. Love is what reminds us we're not alone. Love is what turns pain into purpose. We are all fighting.
But we don't have to do it in silence. And we don't have to do it alone. For those like me lying in a bed day after day, watching life move forward while we remain still there are moments when we feel like a burden. We hate it.
We hate what our bodies have become. We hate needing help with things we used to do without a second thought.
We'd give anything any thing for it not to be this way. And sometimes, we get

angry. But not at you. Not at the ones who stay and love us through it. We're angry at ourselves. At our helplessness.

At the silence of a body that once roared with strength but now refuses to obey. Our world is crashing down piece by piece, quietly, relentlessly and we are forced to watch it happen, unable to stop it, unable to fix it. It's maddening.

It's humiliating. It makes us feel like less. Like we've lost the part of us that was useful, reliable, strong. And God, how we miss who we used to be. We're afraid. Afraid of losing more. Afraid of what's coming. Afraid of forgetting who we are or worse, being forgotten by those we love. Afraid that one day, even you might look at us differently. Afraid of being left behind in every sense of the word. So, on the hard days, when we're quiet or short-tempered, when the frustration shows through the cracks, please, be patient. It's not that we don't love you. It's that we're grieving. Not just the future we won't have, but the parts of ourselves we've already lost.

    Your presence means more than you'll ever know. And even if we can't always say it, we're grateful. We're still here. Still us. Just a little more fragile now. Those like me laying in a bed at times feel they are a burden. They hate their condition they hate being helpless and would give anything for it not to be them. They can be angry but not at you at themselves. Their world is crashing down all around them and there isn't a thing they can do to stop it. It's aggravating and makes us feel worthless and we don't want to be worthless we want to be our old selves. We're afraid, afraid of so many things like losing you and ourselves. On the hard days please be patient.

Chapter Three: What I Leave Behind

Poem: Inheritance of Grit
*"I won't leave gold or silver coins,
No stocks or deeds or business joins.
But I'll leave a story etched in scars,
A compass drawn by prison bars,*

*By courtroom truths and children's fears,
By blood and sweat and unshed tears.
I leave behind a name, not clean
But one my children know stood between
The innocent and all things mean."*

  A man doesn't get to take much with him when he goes. Not the land. Not the house. Not the truck he spent twenty years keeping on the road with duct tape and grit. The things you hold onto the tightest

here. You leave them behind. But the parts of you that mattered
The things you lived for rather than just owned They don't rust. They don't rot. They echo. And I pray mine echo loud enough to reach my children when I'm gone. I've thought long and hard about legacy. Not the kind with plaques or polished boots. I'm not talking about medals or titles. I'm talking about the smell of woodsmoke in a boy's coat when he comes in from the cold.

I'm talking about the sound of a daughter's laughter drifting through the kitchen window while suppers on the stove. I'm talking about the lessons I gave without knowing it the way I carried my burdens, The way I spoke when I was angry, the way I apologized when I was wrong. That's what they'll remember. Not whether I wore a uniform or had my name on the sign. But whether I showed up. Whether I loved them in a way that stuck to their ribs.

   When I close my eyes, I see my boy holding a fish up to the camera, proud as sin. I see my little girl, barefoot in the garden, her dress dirty, but her heart clean. I remember saying things like "not now" or "maybe later." God, what I wouldn't give to go back and change that. To say "yes" to the tea parties. To say, "come here" instead of "give me a minute." Because the minutes run out, don't they? You blink, and the babies are grown. You blink again, and you're the one being tucked in and kissed goodnight. I know now: Time ain't a straight road. It's a loop. And if I've walked mine right, they'll hear my voice in the wind even when I'm gone.

I want to leave them more than photographs. I want to leave them strength. Not the kind that beats its chest. The kind that gets up anyway.
The kind that holds a child through grief, that walks behind a plow, that stands still in the face of loss and says, I will not be moved. I want them to know how to pray not just the words, but the silence in between. I want them to know how to love someone even when it's hard. How to apologize first. How to forgive even when no one asks them to. I want to leave them a map of who I was not just in stories, but in how they carry themselves forward.

I think about the man I was when I started all this. And the man I am now. They ain't the same. And that's a good thing. I used to think dying was about letting go. But I've come to believe it's more about holding on to the right things.

Hold on to kindness. Hold on to faith, even when it doesn't make sense. Hold on to each other. And if you're lucky… hold on to the memory of a man who never stopped trying.

So, what do I leave behind? I leave my hands in the tools my children touch. I leave my voice in the stories they'll tell their own kids. I leave my faith in the way they rise each morning and keep going, even when it's hard. Even when it hurts. I leave them everything that mattered. And nothing that didn't. That's enough. It has to be.

What will I leave behind? I've asked myself that question more times than I care to admit. When the pain gets bad, when the days blur together, when I catch a glimpse of myself in the mirror and see a man, I barely recognize I ask again:

what am I leaving behind? It's not money. That's been gone for a long time.
I spent a year and a half without work before my disability was finally approved and there wasn't any back pay waiting at the end. Thankfully, I'd built up a small collection of Civil War relics over the years. One by one, I sold them on eBay just to keep groceries on the table. Mariah unable to keep a job because she had to take care of me. It was hard and I was too proud to ask for help, hell I still am. Then, out of nowhere, a local church gave me a thousand dollars.
No strings, no questions just grace.
It felt like a miracle. I even took out one of those payday loans, knowing I'd need the cash. Two years later, after not missing a payment, I still owe every dollar I borrowed. I'll probably die still owing it. There won't be any land passed down. No

heirlooms locked in some cedar chest. Just a few guns, the knife I carried in the Army, and a box of memories some of which don't even belong to me. But I'm not talking about things. I'm talking about legacy.

What we leave behind that can't be measured in dollars or divided in a will. Stories. Lessons. Love. That's what I'm trying to leave behind.

    I spent years as a police investigator specializing in sex crimes, mostly involving children. I saw evil. Real evil. And I stared it in the face across interrogation tables, in courtrooms, and sometimes in the mirror on the nights I couldn't sleep. I got a 100% conviction rate for every case that went to court. But no matter how many monsters I locked away, I couldn't save them all.

There are children I carry with me names I've never spoken aloud, faces that still find me in dreams. They were just kids. Innocent, hurting, scared. And I couldn't get to them in time. I forget a lot these days. But not the shoes. I remember the little shoes scuffed and worn,
the kind kids stare down at when they're in pain. Eyes full of fear, but always looking at the ground, like they're trying to disappear. Each pair told a story no child should have to live. And that…. that breaks a man more than bullets ever could. More than disease. More than losing your own mind. It's the weight of what you couldn't save
that stays with you. But I also remember the ones I did help.

    I remember Lisa Miller, and the ladies at the Carl Perkins Center the extraordinary DCS investigators. Strong women. Fierce protectors of children. They fought beside me. They never gave up on the ones everyone else forgot. That place the Carl Perkins Center is sacred ground. Those women, saints. Those ladies, DCS Investigators, Kevin Carter, Roger Rickman they're saints. I've seen them walk headfirst into hell and stare the devil himself down. If you want to see what real hope looks like, walk through their doors.

I hope Riley and Harper know that their daddy fought for kids no one else would. That when I couldn't be there for a soccer game or school function, it was because I was trying to give another child a second chance. I want them to know that being a man isn't about how tough you are it's about how tender you're willing to be when someone else needs you. And I want them to know that I didn't just leave

behind a trail I left behind a path. A path they can follow.
A story they can add their own chapters to. And a name they can carry with pride. More than anything, what I leave behind is love. Not in the form of fortunes or mansions. I don't have those things to give. There won't be a trust fund, or a plot of land, or a safe full of riches. But what I do leave… is something just as lasting, maybe even more valuable. My wife and my kids they'll know how to survive. They'll know how to shoot straight and true,
how to track and hunt and handle themselves in a world that isn't always kind. They'll know how to grow food from the soil, how to fix what's broken, how to face the wild with courage and calm. They'll know the old ways.
How to split wood and read the sky.

How to listen closely and live simply. How to make do with what you have, and take pride in doing things with your own two hands. They'll know the value of hard work, of telling the truth, of standing up for someone who can't stand for themselves. And they'll know they were loved fiercely, unconditionally, without limits. That matters more than anything money could ever buy.

I may not be leaving behind material wealth, but I'm leaving a legacy of knowledge, of resilience, of character. That's what I hope lives on long after I'm gone. Not just in stories told around a fire, but in the way they choose to live.
In how they raise their own children one day. In how they face hardship with strength and treat people with kindness, even when the world doesn't deserve it.

That's my gift. That's my inheritance to them. Love. And everything that love taught me to pass on. If you're laying in bed upset wondering how the family will even pay for your funeral know love is enough. If you're a caregiver let them know the same, remind them money isn't what makes them important.

Most folks think about legacy like it's something big. Land, money, maybe a building with your name on it. But I think they've got it all wrong. Legacy ain't loud. It ain't carved in stone. It's carried quietly in the hearts of the people you chose to love while you were here.

For over 20 years, I've done something almost no one knows about. Every month without fail I paid for a bouquet of flowers to be sent to someone going through a hard time. Sometimes I knew who they were a stranger I overheard in line talking about losing a loved one, a waitress having a rough shift, or a tired mom I bumped into at the grocery store. But most times… I left it up to the ladies at the flower shop. I'd just say, "Y'all find someone who needs a lift this week," and they'd do the rest.

No card. No name. Just petals and color and hope.

I didn't do it for recognition. Hell, part of the charm was in not being known. I wanted those flowers to feel like grace. To show up when someone felt invisible and remind them that the world still had good left in it. That somebody out there cared even if they didn't know who.

Some folks might call that silly. A waste of money. But I'll tell you this I've had strangers break down crying, clutching a bouquet, saying it was the first nice thing that had happened to them in weeks. I've

had a nurse tell me once that an elderly woman received flowers on the anniversary of her son's death and said it felt like a message from heaven.
Truth is, I don't even remember all the stories. But I remember how it made me feel. Like I was still doing something good in a world full of hurt. My favorite flower memory is, I once sent some to a young lady who had been feeling down, when she received the flowers she put a picture of them on Facebook, saying she had received them but didn't know where they came from, some young man took credit for them. They began dating and are now married with children. For $50 I created a family, some may say the relationship was based on a small lie, but I like to think the love was there I just nudged it along.

Legacy ain't always about what you leave for people. Sometimes it's what you leave in them.

I've built things. I've served. I've buried friends and carried brothers through grief and war and heartbreak. But nothing ever felt quite like walking into that flower shop once a month, tipping my cap, and saying, "Let's do another."

So, when I go, and people start talking about what I left behind I hope someone remembers the flowers. I hope they remember kindness that didn't need a name. And I hope they carry that forward. That's what I leave behind.

Chapter 3.5

Still Holding On

The ache of living, the fear of leaving. I don't want to die. Not really. Not even on the worst days. And God knows there've been plenty of those. There are days when the pain swells like a storm inside my skull where my head feels like it's full of water,
like a wave rising from the base of my spine and crashing forward.
It floods my thoughts. It takes my legs, my voice, my dignity.
There've been times I couldn't walk. Couldn't speak. Times I didn't make it to the bathroom.
Times I laid there wet, humiliated, and furious that my body betrayed me again.

And in those moments… yes, I've prayed for it to end. I've begged, even. Quietly. "God, please… if this is all that's left, take me." But those prayers are fleeting. They come in the waves.
And like the tide, they always pull back. Because even in that darkness, there's still a flicker of something in me that refuses to let go. A voice small but stubborn that says,
"Not yet. Not today." I don't think most people truly wish to die. Not even the ones in agony.
We're built to hold on. To cling to this world with torn fingers and shaky breath, because somewhere deep down, we still remember how much it means to live.
  We hold on for small things the way your kid's voice sounds saying "Daddy" the smell of dirt after rain the heat of coffee in your hands when everything else

is cold the dog curled up beside your chair like she knows something's wrong but loves you anyway the simple gift of one more morning, even if it hurts And yeah, sometimes I feel like a burden.
Sometimes I look at the faces around me and wonder if I'm just what's left behind. But even in that doubt, I feel their love. And I hold on. Dying is hard.
But wanting to die that's not as common as people think. What we really want is for the pain to stop. What we really want is to feel whole again, if only for a minute. What we want… is not death.
It's peace.

So, if you're reading this and you've felt that wave that crushing, drowning, shame-soaked tide I see you. You're not weak. You're human. And your fight to stay? That's the bravest thing you'll ever do.

Chapter Four: Memory and the Mind

Poem: Fragments
"Some days I'm here, some days I fade,
Lost in shadows my own mind made.
I reach for names that float away,
And wonder if I said what I meant to say.

Memories flicker, soft then gone,
Like fireflies that won't stay long.
But in this fog, I still can see
The love that somehow clings to me."

Memory is a fragile thing sometimes cruel in what it remembers, and sometimes even crueler in what it forgets. There are days I'd give anything to recall a face clearly, or the sound of someone's laughter that's slipped away like fog at sunrise. And yet there are memories I can't shake ones I'd trade a lifetime to be rid of. I used to pride myself on remembering everything. Details were my job crime scenes, interviews, names, faces, the little tells folks give away when they lie. But the mind doesn't hold up forever, and neither do the stories we carry. Some just fade. Others unravel. it's strange to feel your own mind betray you. To search for a word and find only blank space. To forget why you walked into a room. To look at someone you love and feel the fear that someday you might not know them at all. But what I've learned is this: memory isn't just in the brain. It's in scars and calluses, in how your daughter tucks her hair behind her ear the way her momma does, in the shape of your son's jaw when he's angry. It's in the land, the woods, the creek, the work we do with our hands. You might lose the memory but the love, the impact? That lingers. There are stories etched so deep into your bones, not even time can steal them. Like the first time I held Harper in my arms tiny and fierce, hollering like she already knew the world owed her a fight. Or Riley, barely more than a whisper when he came into this world, now louder than life itself. When I forget what day, it is, they remember. When I lose my place, they guide me back. And maybe that's what family is a lighthouse when your mind goes dark. And let's not forget the mind's stubborn streak. It likes to revisit old wounds when you're trying to sleep. It drags you back to the worst days, the ones you buried. I remember the kids I couldn't save. The cases that haunt me. I remember their names, their faces, their voices when I close my eyes. I carry them. But I also remember grace. I remember forgiveness. I remember being told, once, by a little girl whose abuser I helped convict, that she wasn't afraid anymore. That she slept soundly now. That memory? That one I'll keep.

You don't realize how fragile memory is until it becomes something you have to chase. It used to come easy like breath, like blood. I'd walk into a room and know why I was there. I could tell you what I had for lunch on a Tuesday six years ago. I could trace boot prints through the woods and tell you who made them and how fast they were running. Now I get lost in my own house. Walk into the kitchen and forget what I came for.

Sometimes I leave the water running. Sometimes I forget if I already took my medicine. Sometimes I take it twice. And worse than forgetting is knowing you're forgetting. That ache? That's a different kind of pain. One that settles in your chest and doesn't leave. They don't tell you that memory loss feels like mourning. But it does. Mourning yourself
not the man in the mirror, but the man who used to remember.

The one who could recite case numbers, remember phone numbers from memory, and tell you who made the first pot of coffee at the station each morning just by the taste of it. Now I take notes just to remember who came by.
I write things down and stare at my own handwriting like it belongs to someone else. I've left sticky notes on top of other sticky notes. Sometimes I forget which

ones are old. Sometimes I forget which ones are mine. I've hidden whole conversations from myself.

There's a fear that comes with forgetting. Not the fear of losing facts but the fear of losing yourself. Like little pieces of you are falling off in the dark, and no one sees it happening but you.

You start second-guessing everything. Was I always like this? Did I always have a short temper? Did I really tell her I loved her that day, or did I only think about saying it? It eats at you. That's why I'm writing. Because maybe if I write enough, the words will hold on tighter than I can.

But it ain't all gone, not yet. There are memories that hold fast. Like roots in rock. I remember my mom's perfume White Shoulders like she just walked through the room. I remember my brother

Billy's laugh when he'd talk me into something dumb. I remember Cody's quiet kindness, the way he saw the world without judgment. Like his heart skipped all the parts of life that turn most folks mean. I remember Riley's first deer hunt. The way his boots were too big, but he walked proud anyway.
And Harper, baby girl with wildflowers in her hands and dirt on her knees, telling me I was her "whole heart."

    That's what sticks. That's what I fight to keep. Memory ain't just data.
It's scent and sound. It's the feeling of wood under your hands. It's the sting of cold air in your lungs on a February morning. It's the rhythm of your wife's breathing when you're both half-asleep, and the way she tucks her hair behind her ear when she's trying not to cry. I might

forget what day it is. But I remember love. I remember hurt. And I remember grace.

Sometimes I wonder if people see me slipping. If they notice the hesitation in my answers. The way I repeat myself. If they pity me. But what I want more than pity is understanding. Because this mind of mine? It's still trying. It's still reaching. Still full of stories. And even if I forget the details, the heart of the thing is still here.

There's a grief in knowing my children might one day ask, "Daddy, do you remember when…" and I won't. But here's the thing They will. They'll remember the way I looked at them when I was proud. The way I made breakfast on Saturdays, even if it was just toast and bacon. The way I danced with their mama in the kitchen when I thought no one was watching. They'll carry the best of me forward. Even if I can't carry it myself anymore.

And maybe that's the secret of memory It's not really meant to be hoarded. It's meant to be shared. Poured out like sweet sorghum, thick and warm,
over the lives of the ones, you love. I can't take it with me. But I can leave it behind, slow and sticky, in the hearts of those who mattered most. So, I write this down now while I still can.

I write because I'm scared. Because I'm tired. Because I need these words to live longer than my bones. I write to give my children something to hold when I'm gone. Not just a book, but a voice. A voice that says: I was here. I remembered you. And I loved you until the very last light.

This chapter may not be neat.

It may not follow any rule of structure or style. But that's how memory works. It's crooked. It loops and stutters. It doubles back on itself. And still, still it matters.

So, if you're reading this, and you're losing parts of yourself, I want you to know you're not broken. You're not less. You're just human. Beautifully, painfully, courageously human. And if someone you love is fading Hold their stories close. Say their names often. Write things down. Because even when the mind forgets…the love always remembers.

I used to think memory was something solid. Like a tool hanging in the shed maybe rusted, maybe worn but still there when you reached for it. Turns out, it's more like mist. Some days it drifts in gentle, wrapping me up in familiar warmth. Other days, it vanishes before I can name a face or finish a sentence. And I'll be damned if that doesn't hurt more than anything the body can throw at you. It's a cruel thing, when your own mind starts to slip away. Not all at once, but slow. Like a house settling into rot. You forget where you put your phone. Then you forget a name. Then one day, you're looking at a picture of someone who once held your heart, and you feel panic because you can't recall their voice. I've had days where I find sticky notes all over the house, reminders from myself to myself. Just trying to stay one step ahead of forgetting.

But every now and then God bless it something sticks. Something stays.

I remember being overseas, living out of a damn duffel bag that I couldn't even unpack. Didn't have space. My bag stayed locked in the conex down at the motor pool, and every morning I'd hike down there just to change into a clean uniform. It was a humiliating time, one where I felt like a ghost in my own unit.

That changed the day First Sergeant Fraley pulled me into his office. He didn't say much, just looked at me and said, "You're moving in with the sniper section." Now, that might sound like a promotion, but those boys didn't want me there at first. They were elite tight-knit, sharp-eyed, and skeptical of anyone who hadn't bled with them.

So, I bled.

I volunteered for a makeup ruck march. Twelve miles. Thirty-five pounds on my back. No shortcut, no mercy. I didn't walk it I earned it. I passed within the standard, didn't fall out, didn't complain. And after that, their tone shifted. I could feel it in the way they nodded, in the way they didn't question me so much anymore. They started calling me "the old man," and before long, I was training with them, learning their drills, lending my tracking skills to their mission.

At the end of the deployment, they gave me a sniper section T-shirt. No speeches. No ceremony. Just handed it to me, quiet and honest, and told me "you earned this" That shirt meant more to me than any medal the Army ever gave me. Because it was earned. Because it came from the kind of men who don't give anything they haven't bled for themselves.

Even now on my worst days, when the fog rolls in and I can't remember what I ate for breakfast I remember that. I remember every damn step of that ruck. I remember how that T-shirt felt in my hands.

So no, memory ain't perfect. Mine's broken in places I can't fix. But it's also stubborn. It holds onto what matters. And sometimes, when I close my eyes and reach for something solid, it gives me back the things I need most the weight of that pack, the gravel under my boots, and the moment I was told, without words, "You belong."

And that… that's enough to keep me going.

Chapter Five: The Measure of a Man

Poem: What Makes a Man

It ain't in medals or folded flags,

not in the grip of a handshake firm,

nor the boots worn down by roads marched long

though all of those things have their place.

It's in the firewood cut and left without a name,

the whispered prayer over sleeping children,

the hand that steadies another

when its own fingers tremble.

It's in carrying burdens he never speaks aloud,

in showing up even when the world

has all but forgotten his name.

It's in the moments

no one sees

but God.

A man ain't measured in the battles he wins,

but in the ones, he fights and never brags about.

In what he builds,

what he leaves behind,

and who still weeps when they speak his name.

It ain't medals on a chest, letters after a name, or how smooth a man can make small talk at a dinner table that tells you who he really is. It's what he carries in silence. It's the weight behind his eyes when no one's paying attention, the kind of tired he doesn't talk about, and the way he handles himself when he's got every reason to quit but doesn't.

A man's measure isn't found in the spotlight. It's back in the shadows, behind closed doors, when the crowd's gone home and all that's left is the dull tick of the clock, the ache in his back, and the list of things he said he'd take care of things nobody else even knows about. It's in how he shows up. Not once. Not when it's easy. But day after day, when it's hard. When nobody notices.

It's the way he tightens a bolt just right on something rusted and half broke not because anyone will ever see it, but because he knows it matters. It's the way he checks on folks who ain't checked on him. How he shows up with a chainsaw when the storm's cleared and the roads still blocked. It's the kind of strength that doesn't come from lifting weights but from carrying burdens and never setting them down where someone else might trip over them.

I learned all that without ever needing a lecture. I learned it from my daddy, E.T. a quiet man with heavy hands and a steady heart. He didn't talk about grit or manhood. He just lived it. I watched him haul firewood to folks too proud to ask and too poor to buy their own. He'd stack it neatly, never said a word. Just drove away with that old truck rattling like it was held together with prayer and spit.

I saw him grieve my mama like a soldier burying his soul quiet, clenched, never falling apart in front of us boys. He'd disappear behind the barn some nights, cigarette glowing in the dark, and I knew he was talking to God or to her or maybe both. But he never let that grief pour out on us. He just kept being Daddy. He kept going. He still calls me Pineknot. Says I was tougher than one the day I took a limb to the face out in the woods and didn't cry. But truth is, I almost did. I wanted to. My lip was shaking. My eyes were full. But I saw him arms crossed, face like stone, and something in me steadied. Not because I was trying to be brave. I just didn't want to let him down. That's how boys learn, you know? Watching their fathers survive what would break most men and doing their damnedest to follow suit.

Later, in law enforcement, I met other men who showed me what that kind of quiet strength looked like outside the home. Roger Rickman my compass. A man so steady, so grounded, you could navigate life by how he handled his job.

He didn't flinch. Not at death, not at heartbreak, not even when the whole damn system seemed to wobble. He stood his ground. Always.

Then there was JP hard-nosed, relentless. My double, folks said. Looked like me. Walked like me. Same fire in the belly. But it was his refusal to quit that made us brothers. He never gave up on a case, even when it cost him sleep, peace, or sanity. That man would dig through the wreckage of a person's life until he found what was broken and tried to make it right. I learned plenty from him about work, about pain, and about purpose.

And then there's Mike Shipman. Now that man… he'll never be in any history books, but he sure as hell ought to be. When I got deployed, he didn't just say,

"Let me know if y'all need anything." He showed up. Unannounced, unnoticed, but unwavering. Checked on my wife. My kids. Made sure the water heater worked, and the grass got mowed. He didn't need a thank you. Didn't want it. That's what men do they fill in the gaps without needing to be asked.

Josh Gilbert, Matt Rickman, Nick Inman, Kayla, Alli, Mary Kate, Ron, Tony, Ted Robert, Wyatt, Tommy, Brandon, Jon, Zach, Guy, Beaver, Kaleb Sanders, Michael, Rick and so many more and me, We went to war without a battlefield. We hunted monsters hiding behind courtrooms and bedroom doors. The kind of cases that leave you feeling dirtier than the men you locked up. One night, a bullet found Josh another sadly found Rick. We were in it together. There's a moment, that all our blood mixed, that fire and loss, it burned something permanent into us all. We didn't run. We finished the job.

Me and Michael Gilbert tracked a suspect once so far out in the woods the county dog gave up. We didn't. Caught him, too. Folks asked how. I told them: you don't forget how to read the land. You listen to broken twigs, fresh mud, snapped branches. You feel for movement in your gut. That kind of knowing… it's a gift. And a curse. But it made me who I am.

I've worn a lot of titles soldier, officer, investigator, husband, father. But none of them meant more than being called a good man. That's the one I had to earn the hardest. Because manhood ain't a right. It's not given to you with age or rank or paycheck. It's something you prove over and over again, when the easy way-out whispers, and you don't take it.

Being a man means you carry others when they're broken, even if you're broken too. It means owning your scars, your faults, your regrets, and trying every day to be just a little bit better than you were yesterday. It's showing up when you're tired. Listening when you'd rather talk. Forgiving when it would be easier to harden up and walk away.

Being a man doesn't mean being the loudest voice in the room. It means being the last to leave, after everything's been done right.

And when it's all said and done, when the tools are hung up for good and your boots are left by the door what remains? Not a name chiseled in stone. Not what's in the bank. It's the stories people tell when they think of you. It's the quiet tears you left behind. The way you made folks feel strong, or safe, or seen.

That… right there. That's the measure of a man.

Chapter Six: Carrying the Lost

Poem: The Ones I Couldn't Save
I see them in dreams, in the hush of the night,
The children I failed, though I put up a fight.
They whisper my name with eyes full of trust—
And I carry their memory, heavy and just.
Each one a story the world never heard,
Each silence a scream, each drawing a word.
I carry them not for the guilt or the shame,
But because no one else remembers their names.

There's a weight I carry that no one sees. It won't show up in a scan or X-ray. No doctor can point to it on a chart. No nurse can measure it with a cuff. But it's there Lord, is it there. Settled somewhere deep in my chest, like a second set of lungs that only know how to inhale sorrow.

It's the weight of the ones I couldn't save. For years, I worked the darkest corner of the justice system the part most folks don't want to think about. Sex crimes. Especially the ones against kids. And in that role, I saw the worst of humanity. I saw innocence shattered before it even had a chance to bloom. And I did everything I could. Every ounce of me. Every hour I could stay awake. I poured into those cases.

My record? A hundred percent conviction rate in every case that made it to trial. But you and I both know numbers don't tell the full story. Some of them, I didn't get to in time. Some were silenced before they could ever speak. Some trusted someone else who failed them first. Some were so broken that when I looked into their eyes, I felt like I was staring into a place where God hadn't visited in a long time.

I remember the drawings taped up in the interview rooms crayons used like bandages. Pictures of houses, monsters, crying stick figures. Sometimes they'd draw angels. Sometimes they'd draw themselves as invisible.

I remember the way they'd sit. Small hands folded in their laps, eyes flickering like candlelight in the wind. I remember the silence that screamed louder than any words they could manage.

And I remember gripping those case files like I was holding something alive, something dangerous. Because I knew if I failed it wouldn't just mean paperwork. It would mean pain. Real pain. For them. For their families. For years to come. Some cases stay with me. They ride shotgun in my mind, uninvited and constant. I replay them at night. I think about what I missed. Was there a clue I overlooked? A call I didn't return fast enough. A gut feeling I should've followed.

That's a kind of failure that doesn't scab over. It bleeds slow, over time. Quietly. But I don't speak of these things to draw pity. I talk about them because silence helps no one. These children these broken souls they deserve to be remembered. Even if only by me. Maybe my own pain now, my own slow dying, is part of some divine reckoning. Maybe in bearing my suffering, I carry a sliver of theirs a little longer. Maybe when the time comes and I

stand before my Maker, I can look those kids in the eye and say:
"I tried. I swear to you, I tried. I never gave up on you. Not for one second."
I hope that's enough.
Because until my last breath, I'll carry their names. Their stories. Their pain. Not because I have to. But because someone must. And it'll be me.

   I think often about the soldiers I've known the ones who didn't make it back, and the ones who did, but were never the same. Some lost their lives on foreign soil, boots in the dirt and hearts full of courage. Others made it home to parades and welcome signs but found the war followed them, whispering in the dark, coiled behind their eyes.
It's the quiet ones that haunt me most. The strong ones who cracked without a sound.

The ones who couldn't sleep with the lights off. Who drank too much. Who said they were fine until they weren't. I think of the late-night phone calls I missed. The texts I never sent. The gut feelings I buried because life got busy, or because I didn't know what to say.

And I wonder if I had reached out, could it have changed something? Could a simple "Hey, you alright?" have been the difference? I'll never know. That's the hardest part.

These were my brothers. My sisters. People I'd bleed for. People who, in one way or another, bled for all of us. Now their names are etched in cold stone, weathered by wind and time, but still echoing in my memory like roll call.

And in the quiet of the night, when the world stops spinning just long enough to feel the ache, they come to me. Not in fear. Not to haunt. Just to sit for a while. To remind me they were here. That they mattered. That I'm still here to carry what they no longer can.

And Lord help me, I miss them. I miss their laughter, their flaws, their stubbornness. There's a comfort in the thought of rejoining them someday. Maybe that sounds selfish. But when you've loved people that deeply when you've buried pieces of yourself with them it's only natural to long for reunion. Grief doesn't end. It just changes shape. It becomes part of you. Like a second skin that never peels, only stretches as you move.

I carry them too.

Then there's another grief a quieter one. One no one really talks about. It's the grief of unfinished teaching. Of fatherhood interrupted. I think of my kids

Riley and Harper, and it breaks something in me.

I wanted to teach my son how to sharpen a blade. How to sit still in a blind without fidgeting, how to read the woods like a map. I wanted to show him how to build something that would outlast him not just with hammer and nail, but with integrity and kindness.

I wanted to teach my daughter that strength and softness aren't opposites. That a girl can swing an axe and still cry during a sunset. That she should expect the world to be hard but never let it harden her. I wanted to show her how a man should treat her not just in how I treated her mama, but in how I held her when the world felt too big.

I wanted to leave pieces of myself behind not just pictures, not just stories. "Me."

My voice, my hands, my laugh, my way of watching the sky before a storm.
And it hurts, knowing I might not get to do that.
It's a strange thing grieving your own absence before you're even gone. But that's what this has been. Dying isn't just about the body giving out. It's about letting go of the life you thought you'd have. The years you imagined. The memories you planned on making. It's about learning to love what was, instead of mourning what won't be.
And in that space between holding on and letting go I've found a kind of peace. Not the kind they write about in books, neat and tidy. But the kind you earn through struggle. Through nights spent crying into your pillow. Through days when all you can do is breathe and call that victory.

There are people I wish I'd said more to. Folks who showed up when I was at my lowest. Not with grand gestures, but with quiet presence. A hand on my shoulder. A kind word. Just sitting there in the silence, letting me be. You saved parts of me I thought were gone. I hope you know that. And to the ones I took for granted I'm sorry. Truly. I was tired. I was hurting. But I see you now. I remember.

If there's one thing I've learned, it's this: the smallest acts matter. A hug. A call. A note. A prayer. These are the things that stitch a man back together when he's coming apart at the seams.

And so, I say it plain, before I run out of time thank you. To those who stood by me. To those who forgave me. To those who believed in me when I couldn't believe in myself.

This is for you.

Dedication
To the ones who never made it home
and to those who did but couldn't find
peace once they got there.
To the brothers and sisters whose names I
still whisper in the dark,
whose laughter I can still hear if I close
my eyes.
You were more than uniforms and call
signs.
You were human. You were brave. You
were loved.
And you mattered.
This book, this fight, this breath I take
it's in your honor.
May your stories never be forgotten.
May your battles not be in vain.
And may we who remain
carry you forward
with dignity, truth, and love.

Chapter Seven: Words You Need To Hear

Poem: Words You Need to Hear

*If no one's told you lately
you're doing better than you think.
Even on the days you feel like a shadow,
you still cast light.*

*You're not weak because you're tired.
You're not broken because you cry.
You've carried more than most ever will,
and you're still standing or at least trying to.*

That matters.

If the world's gone quiet around you,

and you wonder if anyone still sees your heart

I do.

I see it in every scar you hide.

You are not a burden.

You are not forgotten.

You are not alone.

You are loved more than you know,

and needed more than you realize.

So, rest if you must.
Fall if you need to.
But don't you dare think
you don't matter.

Because you do.
You always did.

There comes a time when the noise quiets, when the machines hum softer, and even your thoughts slow down just enough to let truth slip in. That's when the final word starts forming not as a speech, not even as a sentence, but as a series of lessons stitched together by pain, grace, and memory.

This chapter isn't just for the dying. It's for those who sit beside us, hold our hands, empty the bedpans, whisper prayers, cry in the shower so we don't see. It's for the nurses who learn our rhythms better than our families, the hospice workers who carry death in one hand and mercy in the other, and the sons, daughters, husbands, wives, and friends who bear the weight no one else sees.

You matter. And this these words they're for you too.

1. There Is No Right Way to Say Goodbye

Let's go ahead and put this one down first: there ain't a blueprint for the end. No rulebook, no checklist, no perfect goodbye. Some people get weeks. Some get a breath. Some never say the words they wish they had. And that's alright. The truth is, goodbye isn't about finding the perfect words. It's about presence. It's about showing up even when your voice shakes or you don't know what to say. It's about being there when the person you love is slipping into that in-between place. Touch matters. Silence matters. Tears matter. Love doesn't need a speech.

If you're the one dying, don't worry about leaving the perfect last words. Just leave honesty. Leave love. Let them see your heart, not your fear. That's enough.

2. Dying Is Lonely, even in a Full Room

One of the hardest truths I've come to learn is that dying, even when surrounded by love, is still something you do alone. No one else can walk that path for you. But there's comfort in knowing people

walked you to the edge and waited, holding your hand as far as they could.
If you're a caregiver, know this: your presence is the light in the fog. Even if we don't say thank you enough even if we're grumpy or quiet or seem far away your presence means the world. Every warm blanket, every sponge bath, every whispered joke, every minute you sit with us in the quiet. It all matters. It all matters.

3. Don't Waste Time Waiting for a "Good Day" to Say What You Mean

People always wait. They wait for the right moment to say, "I love you," or "I forgive you," or "I'm proud of you." But the clock doesn't wait. And dying teaches you this in a hurry: say it now. Say it messy. Say it while your voice shakes. Say it before it's too late.

You'll never regret loving someone out loud.

4. Caregiving Is Holy Work Even When It's Hard

If you've ever washed someone who couldn't wash themselves, fed someone too weak to hold a spoon, or sat in a room where death lingered like smoke you've done sacred work. The world might not see it. There won't be awards. But in the eyes of the person, you're caring for, and in the eyes of Heaven, it's everything.

It's okay to feel tired. It's okay to feel angry, or helpless, or like you're not doing enough. That's love, not failure. Love makes us feel all those things because we're pouring ourselves out drop by drop. So, if no one's told you lately: Thank you. You're a blessing. You're enough.

5. Pain Changes You, but It Doesn't Have to Harden You

There's a choice you'll have to make maybe every day: will this pain make me bitter, or will it make me softer? You can't outrun pain, but you can decide what to do with it. You can use it to recognize pain in others. You can turn it into empathy. Into gentleness. Into strength. Don't let grief turn your heart to stone. Let it carve something beautiful instead.

6. You're Still Here and That Means Something

To the dying: you are still here, you still matter. You still have value, even if your body is failing and your world is shrinking. You're still teaching us how to be brave. Still showing us how to live with grace. You don't have to be cheerful. You don't have to be strong all the time. But please know this your life has meaning right up to the final breath.

To the caregivers: you are still here, too. And that means you have breath in your lungs, which means you still get to love, to serve, to matter. You are not just a background character in someone else's story. You are vital. You are seen.

7. Don't Let Regret Steal What Time You Have Left

Every dying person I've met has regrets. Things they wish they'd said. Places they meant to go. People they meant to make amends with. But regret is a thief if you let it rule you. The only way to quiet regret is to act now. Pick up the phone. Say the words. Write the letter. Forgive. Ask forgiveness.

And if you can't fix it? Then choose to live with peace. You're allowed to let go.

8. Death Is Not the End but a Passing

I used to fear death like a locked door at the end of a hallway. But now, I see it different. Death is a river we all cross. Some of us go early, some late, but no one avoids the water. What I've come to believe is this: it's not the end of the story. Just a page turn. Just a dimming of the light here so it can rise brighter somewhere else.

For the dying don't be afraid. You are walking into something holy. You are not alone. There's more waiting for you than pain. There's peace. There's rest. There's reunion.

And for those staying behind hold tight to the love. It doesn't die. It changes shape, maybe, but it doesn't vanish. It lives in your voice, your memories, your hands. It lives in how you carry them forward.

9. What You Leave Behind Isn't Stuff It's Love

I won't be remembered for what I owned. Most of us won't. But I pray I'll be remembered for the way I made people feel. For a quiet kindness. For the way I told stories around the fire. For the way I held someone's sorrow like it was my own.

The most powerful thing you can leave behind is love. Plant it everywhere. Plant it in your kids, your friends, your neighbors, even strangers. That's the kind of legacy that grows long after you're gone.

10. It's Okay to Let Go

When the time comes, let go. Let go of the fear. Let go of the guilt. Let go of the need to control the outcome. There is peace in surrender. There is beauty in rest. Your loved ones will carry your story. You don't have to carry it all anymore.

Let the ones you love know it's okay to cry. Let them know it's okay to keep living. That you want them to. Let them feel everything grief, joy, confusion, hope. Then let go with grace.

Chapter Eight: Stories I'll Never Tell

Poem: The Quietest Truth
There are stories I'll never write down—
Scenes burned too deep for paper to hold.
They live in my bones, not in books,
Too cruel, too sharp, too cold.
Not for shame—
But because saying them would cheapen them.
Because silence is the only way
To honor what was lost there.

    There are things I've seen that I will carry to my grave. Not because I'm hiding them, but because they're too heavy to share Without crushing the person I'd try to give them to.
Some things you don't talk about not because they aren't important,
But because they are.

Too sacred. Too raw. Too soaked in blood and breath and sorrow.
You see, there's a kind of pain that leaves no room for words.
A kind that carves itself into your marrow,
And if you speak it aloud, it unravels you.
Not in the poetic, redemptive way
But in the kind of way that never gets put back together.
The worst moments of my life are things I'll never fully speak of.
Not to my wife.
Not to my kids.
Not to the friends who would take a bullet for me.
Because I've lived long enough to understand
When you hand someone your trauma,
You're not just lightening your load.
You're placing it on their chest,
And asking them to breathe with it.

And this world's heavy enough already.
I've held dying men who didn't deserve the way they went.
I've heard children describe things they shouldn't have words for.
I've smelled the rot of violence,
Seen the shattered eyes of people who were once whole.
I've watched families implode under the weight of grief.
I've broken, too.
Not the kind of break that makes a sound.
The kind that's silent.
That creeps in at 3 a.m.
That makes you stare at a wall for hours and not remember your own name.
But those stories the ones I'll never speak still shaped me.
They are why I move the way I do. Why I sleep so light. Why I check every door twice and sit facing exits in restaurants.

They're why I sometimes pause mid-sentence, lost in a memory no one else can see.

You wouldn't guess it looking at me. From the outside, I'm just a man. A dad. A husband. A cop. A soldier. I split firewood. I tell corny jokes. I wear the same boots until they fall apart. But under all that there's a battlefield. There are names I won't say, moments I won't revisit, and ghosts I've learned how to walk beside without letting them take over.

And you, you've got your own.

If you've lived long enough, really lived, you've got stories too. The ones that don't get shared around the table at Thanksgiving. The ones that haunt the pause between your thoughts. The ones that never quite leave you alone. They shaped you, too. Made you softer. Wiser. Maybe even kinder.

So, this chapter isn't a confession.

It's a memorial.

To the nights that broke us and the mornings we still showed up anyway. To the trauma we carried in silence because handing it over felt crueler than bearing it. To the invisible weight we lifted without applause. To the moments we survived without ever being okay again.

This chapter is a space for you to set that weight down. Even if just for a page. Even if only in your mind.

You don't owe anyone the full story. You don't have to bleed on the page to prove you were wounded. You survived. And that that is a legacy all its own. The Fear Between the Lines There's something I need to say, something I've held tight to since page one: I was scared I wouldn't finish this. Not because I didn't want to but because I wasn't sure I'd live long enough.

There were days I stared at this screen, fingers frozen, heart pounding, wondering if today was the day the words would die with me. Days when the pain stole my breath. Days when my brain betrayed me, scrambled my thoughts, and left me sitting there, empty, with a blank page and a full heart.

And what haunted me wasn't dying it was leaving without telling the truth. Without getting to say the things that mattered. Without naming the people who kept me tethered. Without handing off the torch I've carried all these years.

If you're reading this now, then I made it. Not to the finish line of life but to the finish line of this story. And that's a kind of miracle I never take lightly.

But still, I carry guilt. I know I didn't name everyone who mattered. I know I forgot stories that should've been told not out of neglect, but because my memory failed me. Or the pain got too loud. Or the words just wouldn't come.

So let me say this now, plain and clear: if you ever made me feel seen, safe, or loved even for a moment you're in this book.

You're in every line I wrote. Every tear I shed while writing it. Every prayer I whispered over the keyboard.

You mattered.

I hope you hear that loud and clear, even if your name's not written here.

Until We Meet Again

If you've walked with me through this chapter, thank you. You've carried a piece of my soul now. And I hope you carry a little of its strength, too.

I didn't write this book for recognition. I wrote it because I needed the people, I love to know what they meant to me before I ran out of time. If I'm already gone when your eyes hit this just know I didn't quit. I didn't forget. I just ran out of time.

So let these final pages be your reminder You don't need to explain every scar. You don't have to tell every story.

You just have to keep going. With grace. With grit. And with the quiet knowing that surviving is enough.

That you are enough.

That even now, even broken, you're still whole.

I'll see you again someday.

Until then… live like it matters.

Chapter Nine: What I've Learned from Dying

Poem: What Dying Taught Me

Dying didn't teach me to fear the dark

it taught me to notice the light.

The way a child's laughter hangs in the air,

or how a woman's touch can still quiet the pain

when nothing else can.

It didn't make me bitter.

It made me honest.

*I learned that silence holds more truth
than sermons,
and that a whispered "I love you"
carries more weight than medals ever did.*

*I found out that peace doesn't come
in the absence of pain
but in the presence of grace
despite it.*

*Dying showed me what matters:
a name spoken with love,
a hand held through the night,*

a life remembered

for how it made others feel less alone.

If I leave anything behind,

let it be this

that you are enough,

that love never dies,

and that we're not defined by our endings

but by the way we showed up

when the curtain began to fall.

Dying teaches you things the living can't quite grasp. It's not because we're wiser or braver it's because time sharpens everything. When the finish lines in sight, you start noticing what matters, and what never really did.

So, I want to share what I've learned not as a sermon, not as a farewell speech, but as a quiet offering. A final handful of lessons scraped together from pain, love, loss, and everything in between.

1. You Can't Outrun Pain, but You Can Make Peace with It

For a long time, I fought the pain. I thought if I stayed tough enough, if I gritted my teeth hard enough, I could outrun it. I couldn't. But I did learn this: you can make peace with it. You can let it walk beside you without letting it lead. Pain teaches you what matters. It strips away ego and nonsense. It makes you look people in the eye and say what you mean.

2. Small Things Are the Big Things

The world teaches us to chase after promotions, money, recognition. But dying taught me that the moments that mattered most weren't loud. It was my daughter's laugh in the kitchen. My son leaning on my shoulder during a movie. My wife rubbing my back at 3 a.m. when sleep wouldn't come.

Don't miss the little things. That's where life happens.

3. Tell the People You Love That You Love Them

Say it. Out loud. Every time. Even if it feels awkward. Say it when they're walking out the door. Say it in the middle of an argument. Say it when they're asleep, and you're wide awake in the dark, hoping for more time.

No one ever says "I love you" too much.

4. Forgive Even If You Never Get an Apology

Holding onto bitterness is like drinking poison and waiting for the other person to hurt. It only eats away at you. I've learned to forgive people who never said they were sorry. Not because they deserved it but because I deserved peace.

Let it go. You don't have to carry their weight on top of your own.

5. Time Is the Most Expensive Currency You'll Ever Spend

You can earn back money. You can rebuild a house. But you'll never get back time. Spend it wisely. Spend it on the people who make you feel alive. Don't waste it explaining yourself to folks who'll never understand. Don't trade it for empty praise or temporary things.

Give it to your kids. To your partner. To a good dog and a slow morning. That's where the gold is.

6. Pride Will Starve You If You Let It

There were times I needed help and didn't ask. Times I was too proud to admit I was scared. Too proud to cry in front of people who loved me. That pride cost me moments I can't get back.

Swallow your pride. Say what hurts. Ask for help. The people who love you will carry it with you if you let them.

7. Dying Doesn't Always Look the Way You Expect

Sometimes it's slow. Sometimes it's cruel. Sometimes it's peaceful. But most of the time? It's ordinary. It's making toast one day and not being able to get out of bed the next. It's confusing. Messy. Beautiful. And deeply human.

Don't wait for a grand moment to say goodbye. Make peace along the way.

8. You're Allowed to Be Angry at God and Still Believe in Him

I've yelled at God. Cussed under my breath. Asked why He let things happen. But I've also felt Him in the silence. In the hands of a hospice nurse. In the sound of my child breathing next to me.

Faith doesn't mean you don't question. It means you come back, even after you do.

9. Most People Just Want to Know They Mattered

That's it. That's the secret. We all just want to know our life had weight that we weren't invisible. That we changed something. That we were loved, and that love left an imprint. So don't hold back. Tell people how they've shaped you. Remind them they matter while they're still here to hear it.

You never know what those words might heal.

10. You Can Live a Full Life and Still Wish for One More Day

I've lived a life I'm proud of. I've seen things most people can't imagine. Loved deeply. Fought for the broken. Made my peace. And still… I'd give anything for one more day with my kids. One more sunrise with my wife. One more quiet walk down the path behind the barn. That doesn't mean I'm ungrateful. It just means love runs deep. And letting go, even when you're ready, still hurts.

So, what have I learned from dying? I've learned that strength isn't about how much you can carry it's about how much you're willing to feel. I've learned that love is the only thing we leave behind that matters. That silence can be holy. That grace shows up in the small things a glass of water, a shared memory, the sound of someone breathing beside you when you're afraid.

I've learned that saying goodbye is an art and sometimes the best you can do is hold someone's hand and not let go until you have to.
And I've learned that even as my body fails, even as the curtain begins to fall, I still have something to give.
These words. This truth. This story.
To you.
Take what you need from it. Leave the rest.
And remember this always:
You're not alone.
You were made for this world.
You belong in it.
And your story isn't over not yet.
Not as long as someone remembers you with love.
Not as long as your name is spoken with warmth.

Not as long as your light keeps flickering in someone's memory.
That's what I've learned from dying.
And that, I believe… is enough.

The Questions That Come With Dying

Lessons, Doubts, and the Things We're Afraid to Ask

When you're dying, silence grows teeth.
It doesn't just sit quiet it gnaws at the edges of your soul.
And in that long hush between medicine doses and distant footsteps,
questions rise like mist off a cold river.

Some are whispered in prayer.

Some stay stuck behind the teeth, afraid to break the stillness.
They come from both sides of the bed
from the one slipping out of this world
and the ones too heartbroken to let go.

But every single one of them matters.

Chapter Ten: When the Dew Settles

Poem: The Last Thing I'll Say

I don't need flowers or speeches or songs,
just quiet.
Just the sound of the wind through the trees,
and the memory of laughter
floating somewhere near the porch swing.

If you're reading this,
then I'm already gone—
but not lost.

Not really.

I've left my voice in these pages,
my love in the spaces between.

Don't cry too long.
Don't wait too late to live.
Hold your people close
and your regrets loosely.

Let the dog up on the bed.
Say the hard thing.
Eat the pie.

And when the sun rises,

think of me.

Not as someone who died,

but as someone

who finally laid down

what he'd been carrying

for far too long.

   It begins with your feet in the dew barefoot, quiet. The grass is cool, and the morning is slow to wake. There's a stillness to the hour, the kind that only comes when the earth hasn't yet decided what kind of day it'll be. You stand there, feeling the weight of your bones, the breath in your lungs, and for a moment, everything holds its place. The honeysuckle is blooming. You can smell it, sweet and old, like memory. Like something your mama used to put behind your ear before church. Like the way a child smells when they've been playing outside all day, skin salted, and sun warmed. That smell that's the beginning of goodbye. Not the kind you say at the door. The kind that doesn't use words. The kind that settles deep into the folds of your soul, like creek water in your boots after a long walk home. There is no fanfare to the end. No trumpets. No bright lights. Just quiet. And the soft rhythm of the world continuing without you leaves rustling, a dog barking down the road, your daughter's laugh echoing faint from the porch. You think about a newborn puppy eyes still sealed, belly warm, breathing slow. The way you held one once, in hands that had done too much fighting, too much hurting. And yet, there it was. Soft. Trusting. Needing nothing but your stillness. That's what dying feels like, in the best way. Like holding something fragile and good and knowing your job is simply not to drop it. You don't see your life flash before your eyes like they say. It's slower than that. Quieter. It comes in flashes not of events, but of feelings the weight of your daughter's hand in yours when she was five, the sound of your son's voice the first time he said "Dad," the way your wife looked standing in the kitchen, backlit by the glow of morning coffee and love that stayed. You remember the nights you prayed and didn't think anyone was listening. You remember the smell of your father's old flannel, still holding the scent of cedar and sweat and something close to grace. You remember your mother's voice, even if the words have faded. The tone hasn't. That never leaves. And you think about the people you couldn't save. Not in shame. No not anymore. But in reverence. As if by carrying their names in your bones all this time, you bought them a second life. You carried the lost. You were never empty, even when you were breaking. The trees don't mourn you. They just keep growing. That's the lesson no one tells you. The world will go on. But it will remember you in strange and holy ways: in a scar on a tree where you carved your name, in the rusted remains of a tool you left behind, in the way your boy ties his boots the same as you did. You were here. You mattered. Not because of medals or ceremonies or the way people cried when you went. But because someone will laugh a little softer now. Hold a little longer. Love a little better because they knew you.

So now, as the sun rises just high enough to stretch golden across the fields, you take one last breath not because you have to, but because you want to. You want to taste the morning one more time. You want to feel it in your chest, like gospel. Like forgiveness. This is not the end. This is just the part where you hand off the weight. To the ones who will carry it next. To your son, who will stand in a field one day and think of you when the wind shifts. To your daughter, who will light a fire and hear your voice in the crackle. To your love, who will keep waking up, even when the bed feels too big. Let them live big. Let them laugh loud. Let them stumble, but let them rise, too. Let this be what you leave: Not fear. Not silence. But a trail of light, like fireflies behind a boy running barefoot through the dark. Let them say you lived. Let them say you loved and when they speak your name, let it be soft Not because they're sad, but because some names are prayers. The dew will dry. The honeysuckle will fall. But what you gave the world That stays. So go on now. Step into the mist. Barefoot. Unburdened. And free. The world is quieter for your leaving, but better for your having been here.

Questions the Dying May Ask

Am I still me, even as I disappear piece by piece?
As muscle fades and memory frays, you wonder
is the soul still whole when the body quits being strong?
Do the parts I can no longer hold onto still count?
If I can't remember the stories, am I still the man who lived them?

Was my life good? Was it enough?
You stop caring about resumes, bank accounts, and who saluted you.
You think instead about your daughter's laugh.
The dog who never left your side.
The people you tried to help.

The ones you failed.
Did I do right by them? Did I love in a way that mattered?

Will they be okay without me?
The dying stop fearing death so much,
but start fearing what comes after they're gone.
Will she know how to change the air filter?
Will he remember how to forgive?
Will they hold tight to the good parts and let the bad one's fade?

Did I say the right things in time?
"I love you."
"I'm proud of you."
"I forgive you."
Sometimes those words slip out.
Sometimes they get stuck in the throat.

Sometimes all you get is a touch on the hand that says everything.

What happens next? Will I be alone?
Even those with strong faith find themselves peeking into the dark.
What's it like to leave the body behind?
Will I be cold? Will I be afraid?
Will anyone meet me on the other side?

Was this pain worth it?
You've fought through more hurt than most will ever know.
Is the lesson in the suffering?
Did someone learn from my struggle not to take life for granted,
not to waste another moment?

Questions the Living May Ask

How do I say goodbye without it sounding
like I'm letting go?
They hold your hand and smile,
but their eyes are begging you to stay.
They say, "It's okay if you need to rest
now,"
even though it breaks their own heart in
half.

What if I say the wrong thing? Or nothing
at all?
They rehearse little speeches in the car
and end up just sitting beside you,
talking about the weather,
or holding silence like it's holy.
Both are acts of love, whether they realize
it or not.

Are they in pain? Are they scared?
Sometimes the dying are too proud to say.
Other times, they just don't want to make anyone cry harder.
So, they smile with heavy eyes and let the medicine speak for them.

Did I do enough? Do they forgive me?
The ones who cared for you the spouse who bathed you,
the child who became your nurse,
the friend who brought supper even when you couldn't eat
they carry guilt like wet wool.
They remember every snapped word, every missed call.
They wonder if you noticed the effort or just the weariness in their eyes.

What does life look like after this?

They're scared, too.
Scared of mornings without your voice.
Of walking past your room and seeing your boots still by the door.
Of holidays that feel more like funerals than celebrations.
They wonder if they're strong enough to build a new rhythm without you.

The Unspoken Lesson

Maybe the greatest truth death ever teaches
is that you don't have to know everything to be brave.
You don't have to say it all right.
You don't have to be perfect.

You just have to show up.
You just have to love clumsily, wholly,
with whatever strength you've got left.

Because in the end, it's not about the answers.
It's about the asking.
It's about the hand you reach for, the story you tell,

the moment you lock eyes and say, "I'm still here."

The Things We Leave Unsaid

A closing letter for both sides of the bed

I don't fear the dark like I used to.
Not since I've walked through so much of it already.
But I do wonder what's waiting for me there
and if I'll know the path when I see it.

I don't need speeches.
I don't want promises.
Just your hand, if you've got one to spare.
And maybe a song, if you remember the one I like.

You ask if I'm hurting
and some days, the pain feels bigger than
my body.
But there's no pill for grief or regret,
and this kind of hurt lives deeper than
bone.

You ask if I'm scared.
Some nights, yes.
But not of dying.
Of leaving behind too many unsaid things.
Of not finishing what I started.
Of you thinking I didn't care enough
when I did, I swear I did.

You wonder if you should've done more.
I wonder if I told you how much you
already have.

What I remember isn't the trophies or the
timecards.

It's you, laughing so hard you had to sit down.
It's the way you made coffee the same every morning.
It's the sound of your voice when you said my name.

We are made of those moments.
Woven from them.
That's what lingers.

So, if this is the end or close to it
let me tell you the only truth that matters:

You were loved.
You were enough.
And I was, too.

A Field Manual for Life

Practical lessons for my kids and anyone walking behind me on this trail.

1. Never ignore a gut feeling.
If something feels wrong, it probably is. Whether it's a person, a situation, or a choice listen to that little voice inside. It's there for a reason.

2. Be kind, but don't be weak.
Kindness and strength can live in the same body. Help people. Hold the door. Speak gently. But don't let anyone mistake your compassion for cowardice.

3. Know how to build a fire.

Not just because it keeps you warm. But because learning how to start something from scratch, to build it with patience and skill, teaches you how to survive and how to believe in yourself.

4. Learn to shoot straight and speak straighter.
I taught you to shoot because it matters to know how to protect yourself and others. But I taught you to speak the truth because it matters even more. Always be direct, even when it's hard.

5. Cry if you need to. Then get up.
There's no shame in breaking down. But never stay on the ground. Wipe your face, stand tall, and take the next step. Even if it's just one.

6. Protect the vulnerable.

I made a career of it. You don't need a badge to do the same. Look out for the quiet kids. Speak up when no one else will. The world changes one brave act at a time.

7. Never stop learning.
Books. People. Mistakes. Listen more than you talk. And ask questions. Smart people ask a lot of questions.

8. Be grateful, even when it hurts.
There will be days that test you mentally, physically, spiritually. Find something good anyway. A sunrise. A dog's tail wagging. The way your kid says "Daddy." Count those.

9. Leave places better than you found them.

Campsites. Classrooms. Relationships. Don't just pass through invest. Make things cleaner, kinder, stronger. That's legacy.

10. Say "I love you." Often. Loudly. On purpose.
People need to hear it. Especially when you think they already know.

You're my legacy. More than anything else.
These words, this book it's just paper. But you… you're the living, breathing continuation of every lesson I ever learned the hard way.

So go live well. Live loud. Live honest.

And when you fall because we all do get up with fire in your belly and love in your chest.

That's what your dad did.
That's what a life well-lived looks like.

Letters of Love

To My Son, Riley

Hey buddy,
If you're reading this, I guess life's
changed in a big way. And man, I hate
that I'm not there to walk you
through it in person. But I want you to
know I'm still with you. Not in a ghost
story way, not in the shadows.
I'm with you in the things you do that
make you proud, in the quiet moments
when you don't know what to
do, and in the way you carry yourself in a
world that doesn't always make it easy.
You were never just a kid to me; you were
my reason. My anchor when things got
dark. The boy who looked
at me like I was a superhero, even when I
felt broken. You gave me something to
fight for when everything
else felt like it was slipping away.

Being a man isn't about being the toughest, the loudest, or the one who wins the fight. It's about standing up when it matters. It's about being kind when it's hard, honest when it's risky, and gentle with the people you. Strength is in your hands, but real strength is in your heart.

You don't have to be perfect, son. You just have to be real. Be the kind of man who makes the world a little better for the people lucky enough to know you. Hold the door open. Shake a man's hand with purpose.

Protect what's right. And never be ashamed to cry when something matters to you.

Take care of your sister. Love your mama with everything you've got. And never forget your dad was proud

of you every single day, not for what you did, but for who you were.
I love you, Riley. Always.
Dad

To My Daughter, Harper

Hey baby girl,
You've always had this fire in you, this spark that could light up a whole room or burn down a forest,
depending on your mood. And I've loved every second of watching you grow into that power. You're strong.
You're smart. And Lord help the world when you set your mind to something.
I know it's going to hurt not having me around. And I hate that part more than anything. But I need you to
know something deep down in your soul: I'm still here. I'm in the wind that brushes your hair back, in the
laughter you can't hold in, and in the fierce way you love people. You're my girl. My heart in human form.

You don't have to be perfect. You don't have to have it all figured out. Just keep that heart of yours soft. Be
bold in your dreams, but gentle with your spirit. Love loud. Forgive when it's hard. And when life knocks you down, because it will, get up like the warrior I know you are.
You' re going to change lives, Harper. You've already changed mine.
And when you're older, and someone tries to tell you what kind of girl you should be stand tall. Remind them
you were raised by a man who believed you could do anything. And you can.
I love you, baby girl. Forever and then some.
Daddy

To My Wife, Mariah

My girl,
There's no way I could write this without
tears. Not because I'm sad, but because
I'm so full of love that it
spills out the sides.
You've stayed when it was easier to run.
You've held my hand when it trembled.
You've laughed at my
dumb jokes, even when I forgot the
punchline halfway through. You've seen
me at my weakest and called me
strong. That's not just love. That's holy.
I didn't always say it right. I got lost in
pain, in fear, in the pressure to be more
than I was. But hear me now,
as clear as I can say it: You were my
home. My safe place. My reason. You
gave me more grace than I

deserved and more love than I could ever repay.
When I go, I know the nights will get quiet. The house might feel too big. And the bed, God, the bed will feel too empty. But I want you to fill that space with the sound of music you love. I want you to laugh too loud at
things I would've rolled my eyes at. I want you to live.
Don't let grief be your only companion. You don't have to carry me forever. I'll always be a part of you, but
you deserve joy. You deserve peace. You deserve a life that still has light in it.
If you ever doubt how much I loved you, don't. You were everything. And if I could do it all over again, I'd
still choose you. A thousand times. In sickness and in health, in life and in dying, you were my greatest gift.

I'll be waiting for you, on the other side of time.
Until then, live. Love. And remember, I'm already proud of how strong you are.
Always yours,
Nathan

To My Dad, E.T.

Dad,
There are things I wish I said more when I still had the strength to stand next to you and look you in the eye.
So let me say them now, plain and true: I am proud to be your son.
You didn't need speeches. You didn't chase attention. You just showed up, every single time. You worked hard. You sacrificed. And you loved in a way that never had to be loud to be powerful. When I was hurting, when I was lost, when the weight of the world sat heavy on my chest, you were there. Not with answers, but with presence. And sometimes that's more than enough. You've carried Cody with a tenderness most people wouldn't

understand. You gave him dignity and patience
when others just saw disability. You never made excuses. You just loved. Quiet. Strong. Steady.
Everything good in me, the part that fights, the part that stays soft, the part that never gives up, I got that from you.
And when I go, I need you to know this: I saw you. I saw every sacrifice, every silent prayer, every time you
stepped in without being asked. And I love you more than I ever said out loud.
You were the first man I looked up to. And even now, you still are.
Your son,
Nathan

To My Brothers: Billy, Jason, and Cody

Billy, you're the oldest, and you've always walked to the beat of your own drum, usually on a Harley. You
taught me not to be afraid of the road ahead. That tough isn't just how you talk it's how you show up. You
made your own path, and in doing so, you reminded me I could too.
Jason, you've always been the one who brought calm into the room. A natural businessman, a people person,
the one who made things work. You've got a gift, brother. One that goes deeper than charm, you make people feel seen. That's rare, and it's powerful.

And Cody, man, you're the heart of us.
The world called you special needs. But I just call you special.
You've taught all of us more about love, patience, and joy than we ever taught you. And I hope you always
feel the pride I carry for being your big brother. You matter. You always have.
Each of you carries a piece of me. And when I'm gone, I hope you'll carry that forward. Not just the
memories but the bond.
We didn't always say it. But I love y'all. I always did.
Take care of each other. Keep your hearts soft. And don't be afraid to talk about the hard stuff. That's how
healing starts.
Always your brother,
Nathan

To My Friends

I couldn't list you all if I tried, and I'd be heartbroken to forget a name. But you know who you are. If you ever showed up for me, whether in a hospital room, at the range, around a fire, or just at the right time with the right words then this letter is for you. You saved my life more than once. Not with medicine or miracles, but with laughter. With listening. With just being there when I didn't even know how to ask. I didn't always make it easy. I pulled back. I got quiet. I tried to carry more than I should've on my own. But you didn't let me disappear.

You were my brothers and sisters in
everything but blood and sometimes,
that's stronger. You knew the pain,
the war, the cost of it all and still chose to
walk beside me anyway.
Thank you for forgiving me when I
needed it. For standing guard over my
family when I couldn't.
For making sure I wasn't forgotten.
I love y'all. I hope I made that clear.
And if I didn't, let this be your reminder.
You mattered to me.
You still do.
And always will.

Legacy Lessons

The Knife I Carried
I still have the knife I carried in the Army. It's not fancy. Just a black-handled fixed blade, worn smooth in
places where my fingers rested without thinking. That knife saw more dirt, blood, and broken gear than most
men ever will. I used it to open MREs, cut seat belts, split kindling, and once to pry a bullet from a wall in Selmer.
It's got nicks and scars, just like me. Funny thing is, I haven't carried it in years. But I still know exactly where it is. I can feel the weight of it even
when it's not on my belt. Because it's not just a tool, it's a memory.

A memory of who I was before the pain, before the slipping mind, before this bed became my battlefield.
Legacy Lesson:
The things we carry say something about us. And sometimes, it's not about the object it's about what it taught us to be: ready, steady, and dependable.

Fixing an Old Chair from a Burned House
After my mama's house caught fire, there wasn't much left worth saving. Smoke and water had ruined most
of it. But there was this old chair, half-charred, busted to hell, and covered in ash. Most folks would've tossed
it. Not me. I spent hours scraping, sanding, and rewinding the seat with 200 feet of rope. My hands ached, my back

screamed, but I kept at it. Because that chair wasn't just wood. It was memories. Her laughter. Her prayers. Her smell still faint in the grain. I made it new again, not perfect, but solid. And now, every time I look at it, I know I didn't let her go completely.

Legacy Lesson:

Some things are worth restoring, even if it's hard. Especially if it's hard. Because fixing the broken can be a
way of holding on to love.

The Deer I Missed on Purpose

I had him in my sights. Big buck. Broad chest. Close range. One clean shot and he'd be down. But something stopped me. It was late in the season, cold and quiet. I watched him pause and look around, like he knew. Like he'd lived
long enough to earn a pass. And for once, I didn't pull the trigger. I just watched him walk away.
That night, I ate leftover stew and didn't tell anybody about the one that got away. It was between me and God
and the woods.
Legacy Lesson:

Just because you can, doesn't mean you should. Sometimes strength is knowing when to let something live.

What My Kids Taught Me About Grace

You think you're the teacher as a parent. And in some ways, you are. But Lord, my kids, they've taught me more about life than I ever taught them.
They didn't care if I walked with a limp. Didn't mind when I forgot something mid-sentence. They loved me
fully, in my strength, and even more in my weakness.
Riley would bring me tools I didn't ask for, just in case. Harper once brought me a peanut butter sandwich and

whispered, don't give up, Daddy. I hadn't said a word to her about feeling low. But she knew. They forgave when I was impatient. They hugged me when I was ashamed.

Legacy Lesson:

Grace isn't something you earn. It's something given. Freely. Especially by the ones who love you most.

The Fear Between the Lines

There's something I need to say, and it's been sitting in my chest since I started writing this book:

I was afraid I wouldn't finish.

Not because I didn't want to—but because I didn't know if I'd live long enough.

There were days I was too weak to write. Days my hands didn't work. Days I stared at a blank screen, knowing I had more to say but not enough time to say it. And in those moments, I worried—worried that this would die with me.

That these words... this message... this legacy... would be lost inside a file, never opened, never printed, never read.

So, if you're holding this now if it made it into your hands then that alone is a miracle. That means I made it. Maybe not to the finish line of life... but to the finish line of this.

But even then, I carry guilt.

I know I didn't say everything.

I know there are people I didn't name who meant the world to me.

I know there are stories I left out not because they didn't matter, but because my mind failed me, or the pain got too loud, or the words just wouldn't come.

To those people... I hope you know.

You mattered.

Maybe you were just a kid who held a door when I was struggling to walk.

Maybe you were a nurse who wiped my forehead when I couldn't speak.

Maybe you were a friend from years ago who said one kind thing that stuck.

Maybe you were family, even if we didn't always know how to say "I love you" right.

Whoever you are if you wonder whether you left a mark on me, let me tell you: You did.

You mattered more than you know.

And if you ever doubt that read between the lines of this book. It's there. Every bit of my heart, spread out in these pages. I just hope you can feel it.

I wrote this with urgency. Not because I was afraid of dying… but because I was afraid of leaving without telling the truth.

Afraid that the people I love wouldn't know just how fiercely I loved them.

Afraid the ones who felt small wouldn't realize how big of an impact they had on me.

Afraid my silence would speak louder than my soul ever could.

But this book is my voice. And it is not silent.

So, if you're reading this now hear me:

You were seen. You were loved. You are part of my story.

And if I'm already gone by the time your eyes hit these words, just know…

I didn't quit.
I didn't forget.
I just ran out of time.

Until We Meet Again
If you've made it this far, thank you.

Thank you for walking this path with me step by painful, hopeful, beautiful step. I didn't write this book to be remembered as some hero. I wrote it to make sure the people I love knew exactly what they meant to me.

And if you're one of them if my blood runs in your veins, or if our lives crossed for even a moment, I hope you carry something from these pages with you.

Maybe it's strength.
Maybe it's comfort.

Maybe it's just the reminder that even when someone is gone… their love can stay.

I hope my kids remember how I laughed.

I hope my wife remembers how I looked at her when she wasn't watching.

I hope my friends remember the fire I had left in me, even near the end.

And I hope you, dear reader, remember this:

Life is hard, but it's not empty.

There's purpose in the pain.
There's grace in the goodbye.
And there is still love left in this world for you.

So go live boldly.

Forgive freely.

Love without keeping score.

And if you ever wonder what I'd say to you in your hardest moment…

Here it is:

You're not alone. You're never alone. And you are so much stronger than you think.

I'll see you again on the other side.

Until then, live like it matters.

Because it does.

And you do.

Songs from the Other Side

A collection of poems written in the long shadow of dying, in the quiet hours when pain speaks loudest and memory becomes a lantern.

Son of My Blood

You came into this world fists clenched, like you already knew Life was a fight worth showing up for. You didn't cry loud Just looked at me, like you recognized something Old in my eyes. Something tired but still trying.

You are the arrow I pulled from my own chest and aimed at a better world. I see myself in your stubbornness, Your fire, Your questions about everything.

Son, I don't know how long I'll be able to walk beside you, but know this: Every step you take, I'll be there. Not in the wind or some poetic mist in your grit. In your sense of justice. In the way you carry the people you love.

You were never meant to follow my footsteps. You were meant to go farther.

And if you ever doubt yourself, just remember:
You were born with clenched fists
Because you were ready to hold the world and not let go.

Little Hands, Mighty Heart

You always held my hand Like you were holding the whole world together. Sticky fingers, wild hair, And a heart too big for your chest.
You taught me softness in a life built on steel. Your giggles broke through pain That medicine couldn't touch.
Harper, I wish I could stay longer. I wish I could dance with you at your wedding, fix your car, tell off the first boy who breaks your heart.
But if I can't do those things Let this be enough: You were my joy When nothing else made sense. You made me laugh When my body forgot how.
When I'm gone, don't look for me in the stars. Look for me in the things I taught you How to fix something that's broken.

How to speak truth, even when your voice shakes. How to be fierce, and still kind. Little hands, Mighty heart.
You changed me.

What Love Looks Like

*It looks like quiet dinners with your hand on mine. It looks like holding me When I couldn't hold myself.
It looks like patience Real, gritty patience The kind that shows up When romance fades and reality hurts.
It looks like knowing When to fight, when to be still, and when to just sit beside me While I fall apart.
Mariah, you loved me in the trenches of war, of sickness, of sorrow. And I need you to know…
I saw you.
I saw every time you bit your tongue. Every time you smiled when it hurt. Every time you stayed, even when I made it hard.
This book exists Because of your love.*

If anyone ever asks me what love looks like, I'll tell them: It looks like you.

This Pain I Carry

This pain I carry isn't always seen, it hides beneath the skin, between the words, it smiles through the ache, talks through the cough, And limps through the day as though nothing's wrong. But at night, when no one's watching, it sits heavy on my chest, And I wonder if the weight of it Might one day crush me before the dying ever does.

Silent Battles

The loudest battles I've ever fought Were the ones no one heard. No guns, no shouting just the slow erosion of hope, of strength, of time. And yet I showed up, day after day, To the war inside my own skin. And if that's not bravery, then maybe we need a new word for it.

Inheritance of Grit

I come from men who worked with broken hands, and women who loved through broken hearts. We didn't always have much, but we had grit in the marrow and kindness sewn into every scar. I leave anything behind, let it be that: A legacy of tenderness, built on a spine of stone.

Fragments

Some days I am all memory. Other days, all ache. But even in pieces, I still recognize myself in my daughter's voice, in my son's stubborn streak, In the way they walk barefoot in the grass Like they were born from the land itself. I may be fading, But I am not gone.

Footprints in Clay

We don't get to choose what remains. But sometimes it's the quiet things: The swing creaking in the yard, the boots by the door, the smell of pipe tobacco still caught in old shirts. Footprints in clay. Soft. Shallow. Enough to know we were here.
The Ones I Couldn't Save
There are names I don't speak aloud. Faces that come back in dreams. Little hands, little voices, broken truths. I tried. God knows I tried. But some battles aren't ours to win. Still, I carry them all Not as failure, But as reason.

One More Sunrise

If I could steal just one more sunrise, I'd sit in the dew and let it warm my bones. Not to escape the dying, but to say thank you for the living. Thank you for my children's laughter, For the smell of earth after rain, For the chance to be a man Who felt it all and loved through it anyway.
When I Am
When I am ash, let me be scattered in the woods that knew my name. Let me rest in the riverbed Where I skipped rocks and found God. When I am gone, don't visit a stone Visit the dirt under your fingernails. That's where I'll be. In sweat. In sun. In song. Still here. Still yours.

Ghost in the Darkness

*Cold blue steel in my mouth,
head and heart full of doubt.
Feeling so mad, hurting so bad
there is a ghost in the darkness.*

*He waits for me in the silence,
feeds on every crack in my soul.
Whispers in my ear when no one's watching,
"It'd be easier if you just let go."*

*But I don't.
Not because I'm not tired.
Not because the weight has lessened.
But because somewhere,
there's still a reason to stay.*

My children's laughter.

The smell of rain on fresh-cut fields.
The memory of a woman who still sees me
even when I can't see myself.

I've danced too close to the edge.
Felt the chill of the barrel.
And still I live.
Still, I rise.

Some ghosts don't want to be banished.
They just want to be heard.
So, I listen, and I write,
and I let them bleed onto paper
instead of letting them bury me.

I carry the ghost,
but I carry hope, too.

And that's the end, thank you for joining me on this journey. I want you to understand there were so many more people I wanted to include, so many more stories, from work to melted birthday cakes, I wanted to include, but I couldn't. The headaches from staring at a screen the constant battle with pain. Please know you are important I love you, while your name might not have found itself on these pages it is certainly written upon my heart. I am grateful for you and love you in ways you'll never know.

    To the stranger reading this, know I prayed for you. I feel you, and you've never alone. Your life means something. Tell those around you how you feel, let them know the impact they have had on your life, and how much you love them.

Until we meet again, never give up hope, never give up love! And remember there is a lesson in dying!
    In The Heart, NCH

Made in the USA
Columbia, SC
10 July 2025